AF350227

EMBRYOLOGY
Made Easy

Crash Course for Medical and Nursing Students

Sivajith P R

3d year medical student in government medical
college Kollam, Kerala, India

Published by

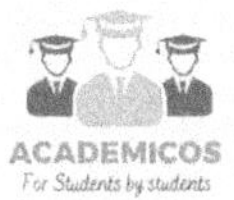

Academicos

Copyright @ Sivajith P R
Contact us: teamwolfrum123@gmail.com

Copyright © 2022 SIVAJITH PR

All rights reserved
No part of this book may be reproduced, or stored in a retrieval system, or transmitted in any form or by any means, electronic, mechanical, photocopying, recording, or otherwise, without express written permission of the publisher.

Dedicated to
My Parents, Brother and Friends

Preface

This book aims at improving the understanding of different aspects in embryology through simple notes and perfect diagrams. This is a small piece from the big world of embryology which makes the identification and studies easier from an examination point of view. This book will help you in covering almost all the essential topics that have been frequently asked in exams. _Let the knowledge spread. _Sharing is caring_
With regards,
Sivajith P R
17/10/2022

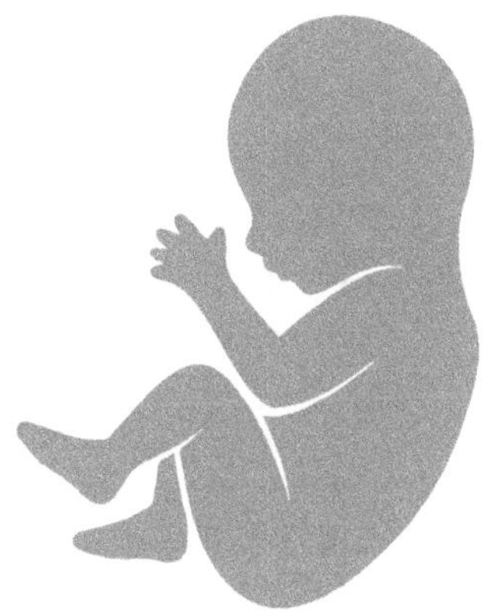

Table of contents

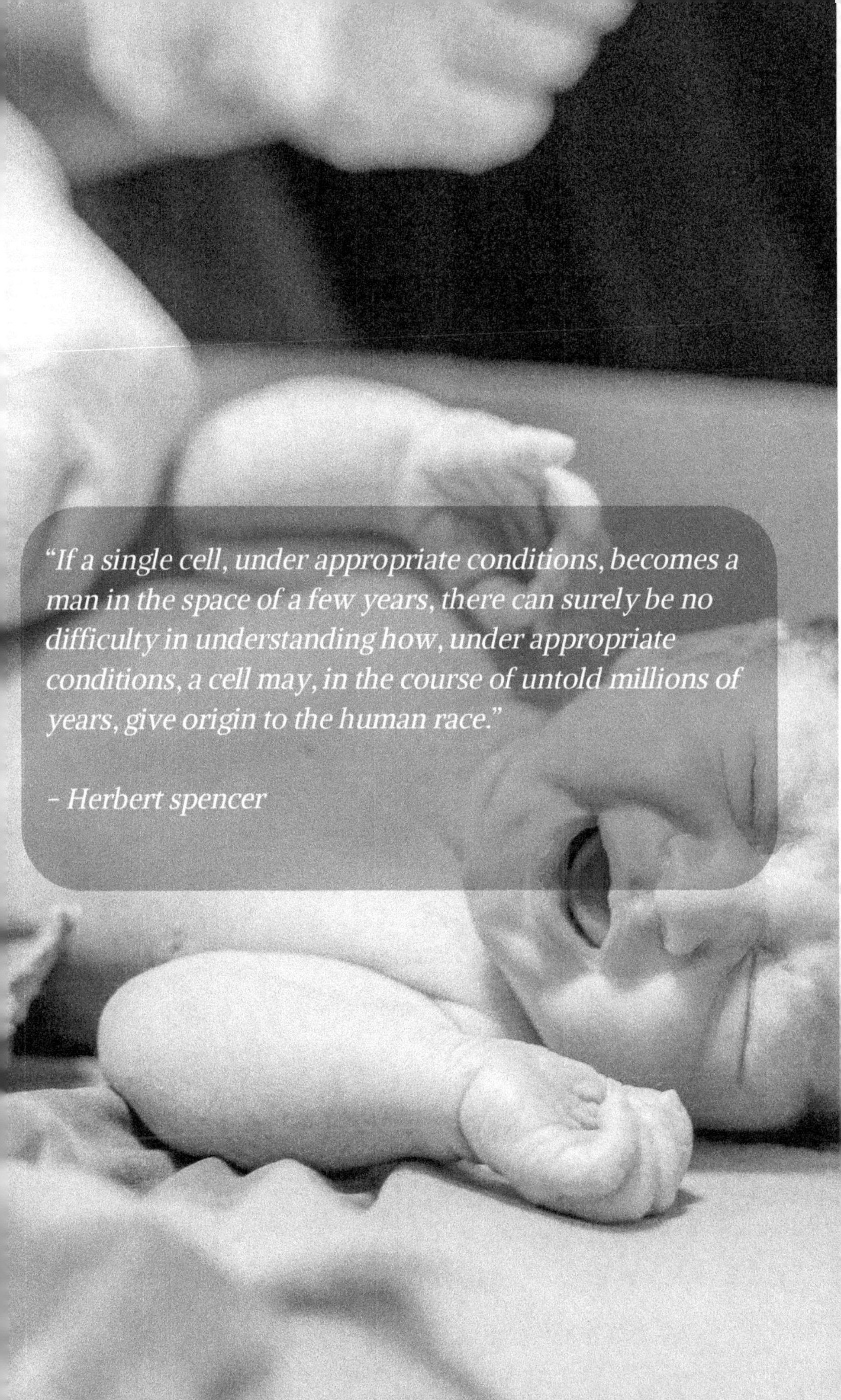

"If a single cell, under appropriate conditions, becomes a man in the space of a few years, there can surely be no difficulty in understanding how, under appropriate conditions, a cell may, in the course of untold millions of years, give origin to the human race."

- Herbert spencer

Introduction to embryology

Embryology is the science that deals with the development of an individual within the uterus. Human development begins with fertilization, which results in the formation of diploid zygote. Human development can be classified into two stages
1) Prenatal development
2) Postnatal development
Prenatal stage is a period which lasts from fertilization to birth. Postnatal stage extends from birth to about 25 years of age
The prenatal development can be subdivided into 3 stages
a) Pre Embryonic period (extends from conception to the end of second week)
b) Embryonic period (extends from third week to end of eight week)
c) Fetal period (extends from 9th week to birth)

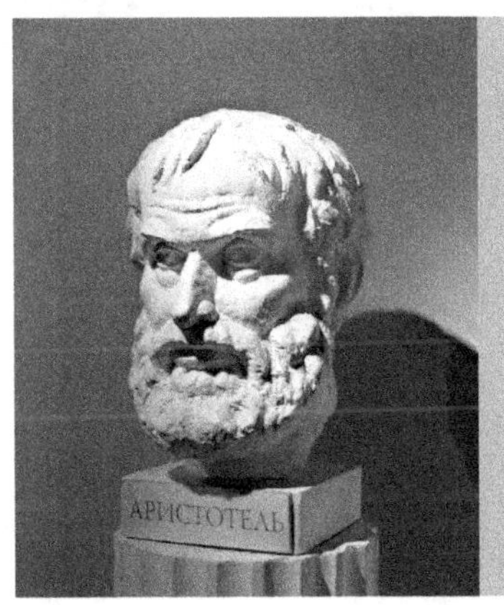

Aristotle is regarded as the "Father of Embryology".He was the first embryologist to describe the development and reproduction of many kinds of organism in his book titled "Degenerative Animalium".

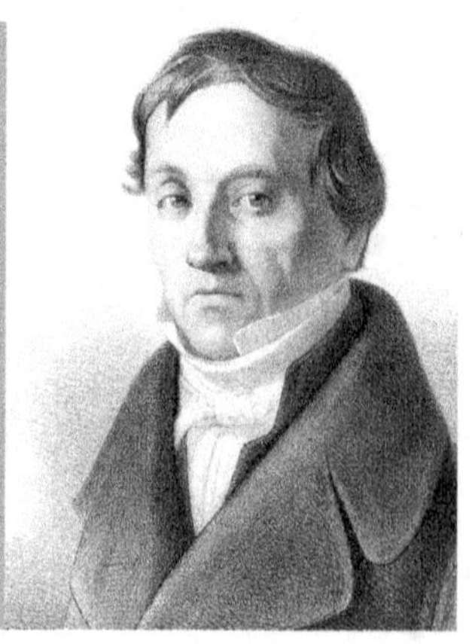

Karl Ernst Von Baer is the father of Modern Embryology. He was born in Russia in 1792. He studied the embryonic development of animals, discovering the blastula stage of development and the notochord.

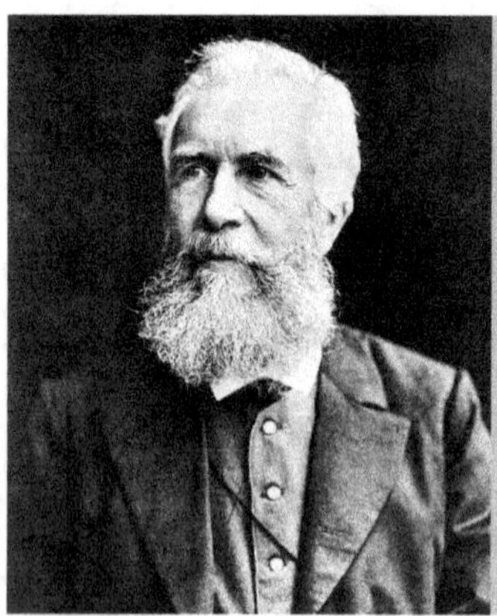

Ernst Haeckel was a German zoologist. He proposed the theory of recapitulation. According to this theory, in developing from an embryo to an adult, animals go through stages resembling or representing successive stages in the evolution of their remote ancestors; thus, suggesting their evolutionary roots.

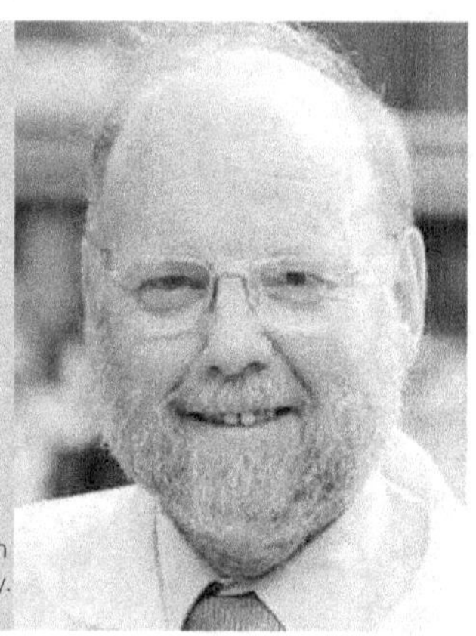

Sir Ian Wilmut, is an English embryologist
He is best known as the leader of the research group that in 1996 first cloned a mammal from an adult somatic cell, a Finnish Dorset lamb named Dolly.

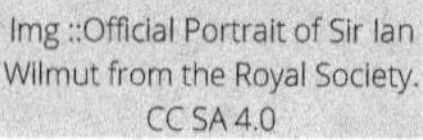

Img ::Official Portrait of Sir Ian Wilmut from the Royal Society. CC SA 4.0

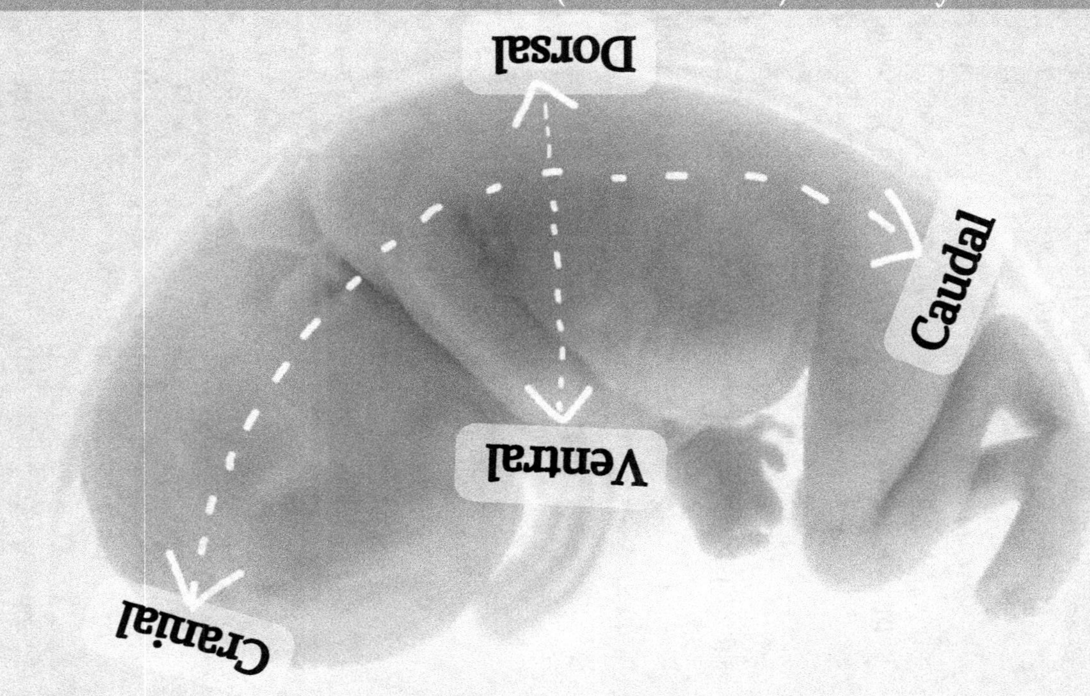

- Ventral: Anterior part (front) of embryo
- Dorsal : posterior part (back) of embryo
- Cranial/Cephalic : refers to head end of embryo
- Caudal: refers to tail end (inferior end) of embryo

Spermatogenesis

- Spermatogenesis is the process of formation of spermatozoa from primordial germ cells (spermatogonia)
- Spermatogonia undergo mitotic division to form two dark type-A spermatogonia
- Each dark type-A spermatogonia undergoes mitosis to form one dark-A type spermatogonia and one light-A type spermatogonia
- Dark type-A spermatogonia are kept in reserve and light-A type spermatogonia undergo mitosis to form two dark type-B spermatogonia
- B-type undergoes mitosis to form two primary spermatocytes
- The primary spermatocytes undergo Meiosis-I to form secondary spermatocytes. Secondary spermatocytes undergo Meiosis-II to form spermatids

Spermiogenesis

- It is the process by which spermatids are transformed into mature spermatozoa.

- Spermatids (immature sperms) are more or less circular cells containing nucleus, golgi apparatus, centrosome and mitochondria.
- Spermiation consist of following sequence of events:
- Nuclear material (chromatin) of spermatid condenses and nucleus move towards one pole.
- Golgi apparatus forms acrosomal cap which covers two thirds of the nucleus.
- Centrosome divides into two centrioles. One becomes spherical and moves towards the posterior end of the nucleus to occupy the neck region . It gives rise to axial filament. Other moves away from the first centriole and form "Annulus" around the distal end of mid-piece

- The part of the axial filament between neck and annulus becomes surrounded by mitochondria and together they form middle piece of sperm.
- Remaining part of the axial filament elongates to form the principal piece and end piece (tail)

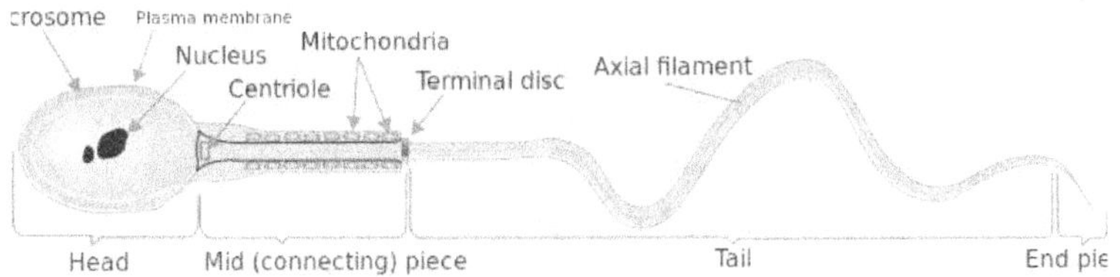

Img[1]: Human spermatozoa copyright Mariana Ruiz Villarreal

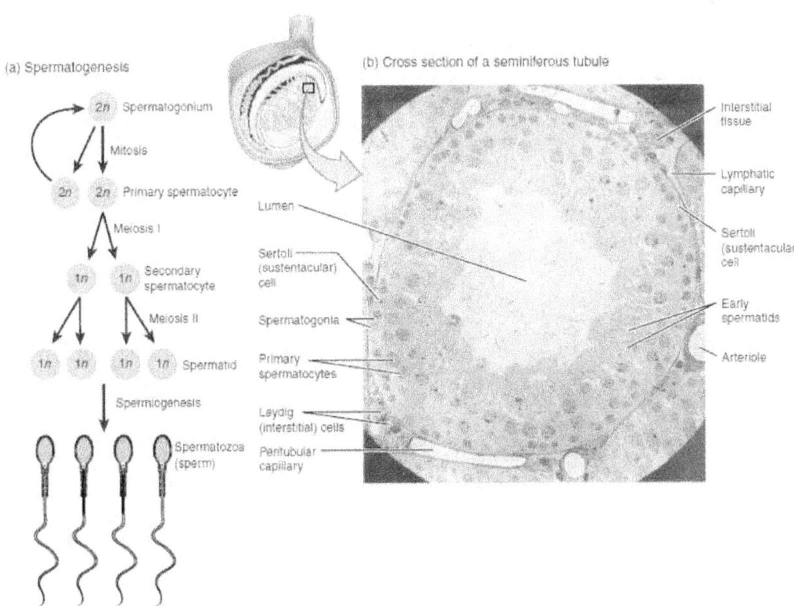

Img[2]: The process of spermatogenesis as the cells progress from primary spermatocytes, to secondary spermatocytes, to spermatids, to Sperm. Image credit OpenStax College • CC BY 3.0 (Illustration from Anatomy & Physiology, Connexions Web site. http://cnx.org/content/col11496/1.6/, Jun 19, 2013.)

Oogenesis

- It is the process of formation of female gametes from primordial germ cells (PGCs).
- The process of oogenesis begins long before the birth, in the cortex of the ovary.
- The PGCs undergo mitosis to form a large number of oogonium.
- Each oogonium enlarges to form a primary oocyte.
- Primary oocyte enters into Meiosis-I.
- But this division is arrested till puberty due to the presence of oocyte maturation inhibitors.
- In puberty the primary oocyte completes Meiosis-I and gives rise to Secondary oocyte and First Polar Body.
- Secondary oocyte undergoes Meiosis-II and give rise to Mature Ovum and Second Polar Body.
- NOTE: Secondary oocyte should undergo fertilization to complete Meiosis-II to form mature ovum.

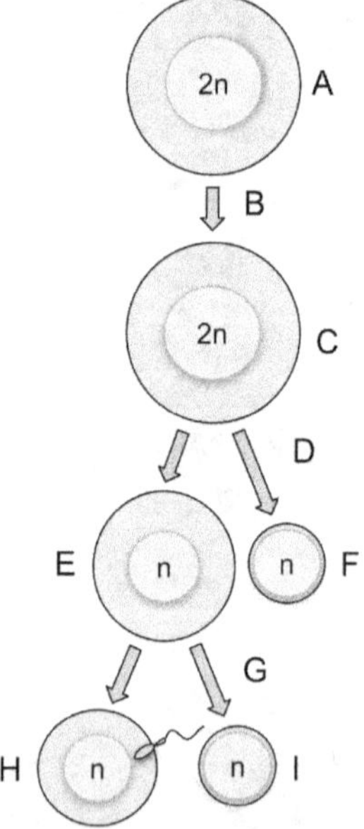

Img[3]:(A) oogonium where the mitotic division occurs (B) differentiation and meiosis I begins (C) primary oocyte (D) meiosis I is completed and meiosis II begins (E) secondary oocyte (F) first polar body (G) ovulation must occur and the presence of the sperm penetration (fertilization) induces meiosis II to completion (H) ovum (I) second polar body _img credit: Leiladavids • CC BY–SA 4.0

Fertilization

Human life begins with fertilization. It is a process in which male gamete fuses with female gamete to form zygote. This zygote undergoes mitotic division or cleavage to form smaller cells. These smaller cells are called blastomeres. Sixteen celled stage of zygote is called morula. In the morula blastomeres are small and are enclosed by a membrane called Zona pellucida. This morula now enters into the uterine cavity. In the uterine cavity the endometrial fluid penetrates the zona pellucida layer of the morula and results in the formation of a cavity called blastocoele. At this stage the morula is called blastocyst. Within the blastocyst the blastomeres undergo rearrangements to form two cell groups

1) Inner cell mass – develops into human embryo

2) Trophoblast – develops into extraembryonic membranes

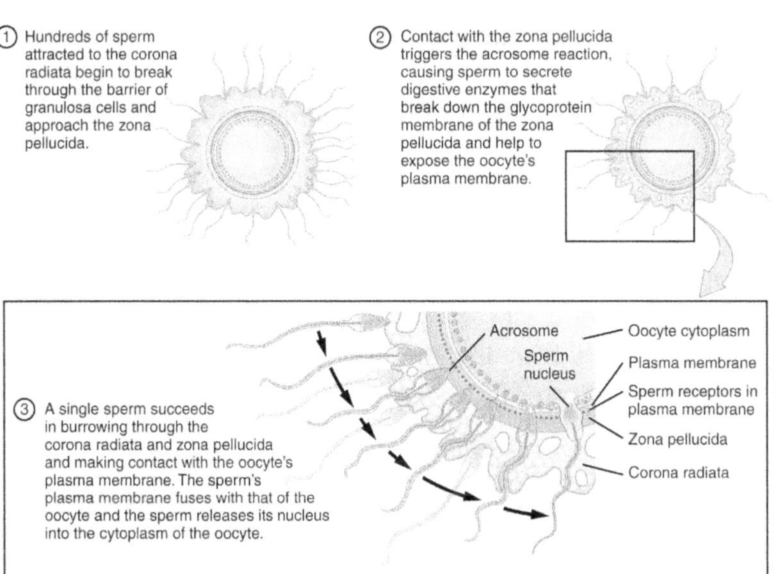

Img[4]: credit _"OpenStax AnatPhys fig.28.2 – Sperm Fertilization – by OpenStax, license: Creative Commons Attribution. Source: book 'Anatomy and Physiology', https://openstax.org/details/books/anatomy-and-physiology.

Blastocyst

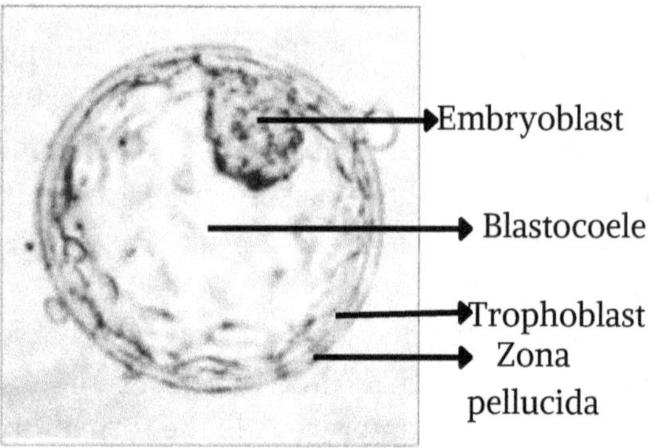

Implantation

- It is the process by which an embryo is embedded and fixed in uterine endometrium.
- Normal site of implantation– upper part of posterior wall of uterine cavity.
- Blastocyst surrounded by zona pellucida enters the uterus on the 6th day
- As the blastocyst enlarges, zona pellucida disappears and trophoblast exposes
- Trophoblast divided into inner cytotrophoblast and outer syncytiotrophoblast
- Syncytiotrophoblast invades endometrium with the help of proteolytic enzymes

- After the implantation of blastocyst, the functional layer of endometrium of uterus is termed as "decidua"
- The endometrium of the uterus will be in the secretory phase (refer menstrual phase) at the time of implantation. After the embryo is implanted, the Syncytiotrophoblast starts secreting HCG hormone.

Gastrulation

Inner cell mass undergoes a series of changes and is converted into a triple layered disc like structure called embryonic disc. The process of formation of tripled layered embryonic disc is called gastrulation

Gastrulation involves following steps:

- Inner cell mass (embryoblast) undergoes differentiation to form two layers: a superficial layer consisting of flat cells called Endoderm (Hypoblast) and a deep layer consisting of columnar cells called Ectoderm (Epiblast)
- Now the ectoderm forms a linear thickening in the midline of the embryonic disc called the primitive streak. At the cranial end of the primitive streak, the cells proliferate and give rise to a rounded elevation called Primitive node / Hensen's Node
- Now a small cavity appears between Ectoderm and Trophoblast, which is called amniotic cavity
- The cells of the ectoderm proliferate and line the blastocoele. The blastocoele now known as primary yolk sac
- The cells of trophoblast undergo proliferation and give rise to mass of cells called extraembryonic mesoderm
- Extraembryonic celom divides extraembryonic mesoderm into

    1. Somatopleuric layer – it lines trophoblast
    2. Splanchnopleuric layer – it lines yolk sac

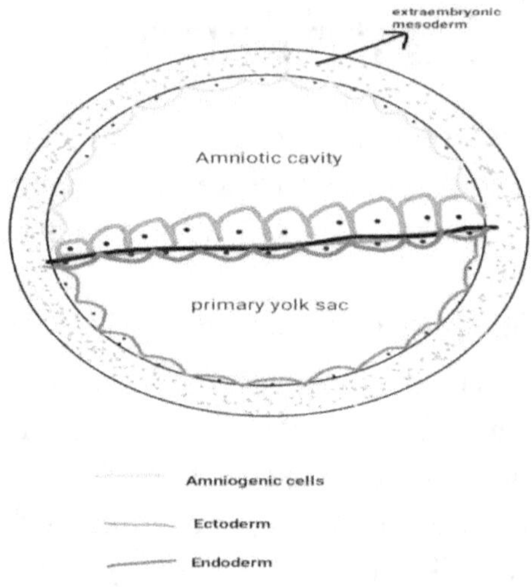

Img: Hand drawn diagram of bilaminar germ disc

- The extraembryonic coelom does not extend into the cranial part of extraembryonic mesoderm, that lies between amniotic cavity and trophoblast. This part forms connecting stalk
- Amniogenic layer + Somatopleuric layer of extraembryonic mesoderm give rise to "Amnion"
- Trophoblast + Somatopleuric layer of extraembryonic mesoderm give rise to "Chorion"

FORMATION OF INTRAEMBRYONIC MESODERM

- A depression appears in the center of primitive node is called blastopore
- A solid cord of cells grow cranially from the bottom of blastopore, between ectoderm and endoderm to the prechordal plate

- This solid cord of cells give rise to a cylindrical structure called notochord
- The cells of the primitive streak invaginates towards the endoderm forming a groove called Primitive groove
- From the bottom of this groove cells of primitive streak spread in between ectoderm and endoderm to form intraembryonic mesoderm
- The intraembryonic mesoderm extends all over the embryonic disc except in certain regions, they are;

1. Region of Prechordal plate – develops into buccopharyngeal membrane
2. Region of Cloacal membrane – develops into rectum and anal canal
3. Region of notochord

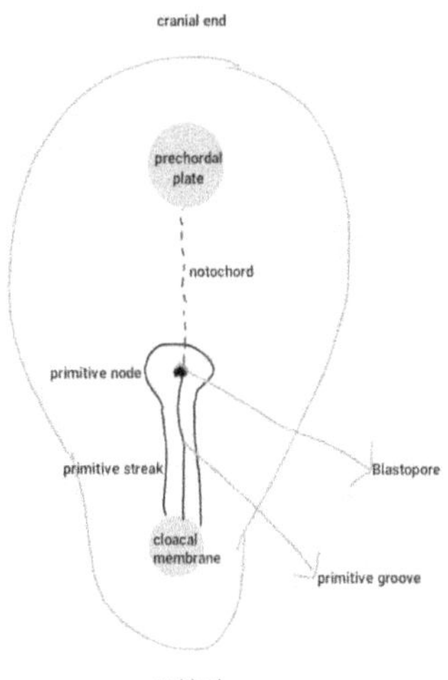

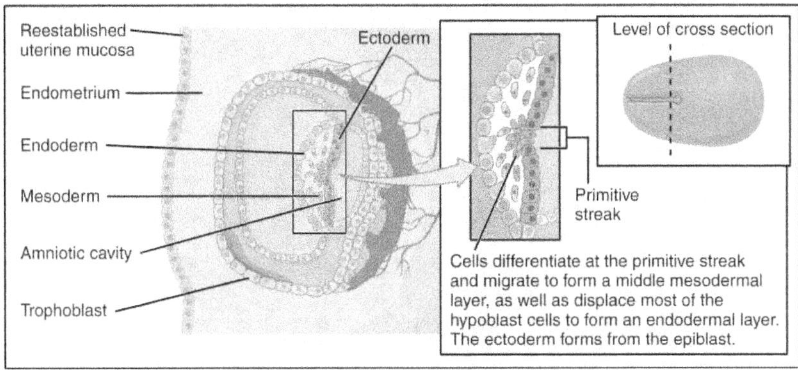

Img[5]: development of mesoderm – copyright _By openstax CC BY SA 4.0] via wikimedia commons

Derivatives of germ layers

Endoderm	• Epithelial lining of digestive and respiratory tracts, • Lining of urethra, bladder and reproductive System • Liver and pancreas
Mesoderm	• Notochord • Musculoskeletal system • Muscular layer of stomach, intestine etc • Circulatory system
Ectoderm	• Epidermis of skin • Cornea and lens of eye • Nervous syst em

Extraembryonic membranes

Extraembryonic membranes or fetal membranes are structures which are derived from zygote but do not participate in embryo formation. They includes

1. Placenta
2. Amnion
3. Yolk sac
4. Chorion

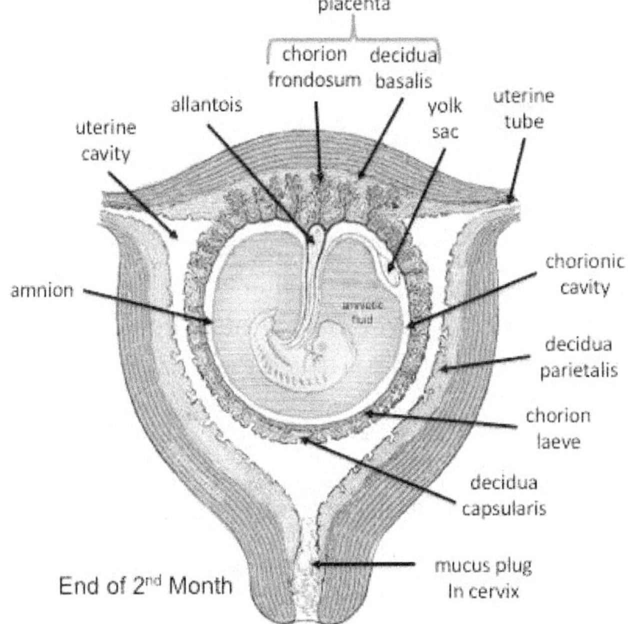

Img[6]: extraembryonic membranes _image credit :Dennis M DePace, PhD, CC SA 4.0 via wikimedia

Chorion

- Chorion consist of Trophoblast and somatopleuric mesoderm
- During implantation the Trophoblast differentiated into cytotrophoblast and syncytiotrophoblast.
- This syncytiotrophoblast rapidly grows and erodes the decidua basalis and becomes thicker.
- Small cavities called Lacunae appear in the thickened syncytiotrophoblast.
- These lacunae increase in their size and are filled with maternal blood and secretion. Now they are called intervillous spaces.
- The part of syncytiotrophoblast which separates lacunae is known as Trabeculae.

Development of chorionic villi

- The cytotrophoblast forms finger-like projections that invade the trabeculae in its center.
- This finger-like projection of cytotrophoblast surrounded by syncytiotrophoblast is called Primary villi.

- The mesodermal core penetrates the primary villi to form secondary villi.
- Fetal blood vessels develop in the mesoderm of secondary villi to form Tertiary villi.
- Tertiary villi forms anchoring villi.
- Anchoring villi: Villi which are attached to the decidua is anchoring villi. Usually it will be a tertiary villus.
- Floating villi: Villi which is floating in the maternal blood is called floating villi.

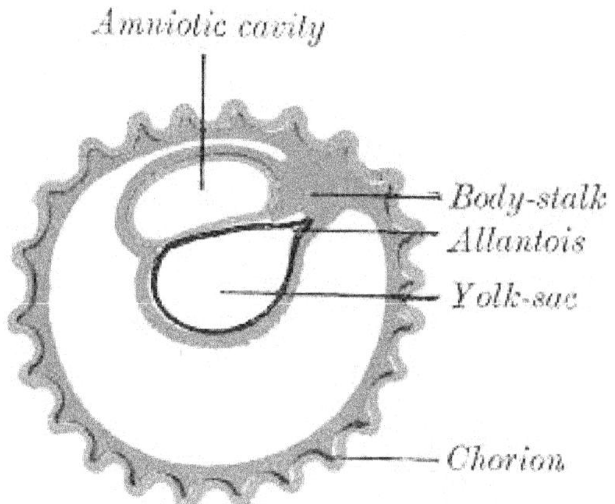

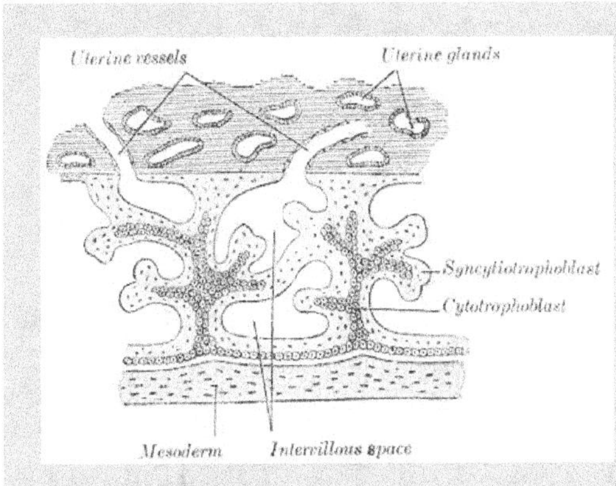

Primary villi

Tertiary Villi

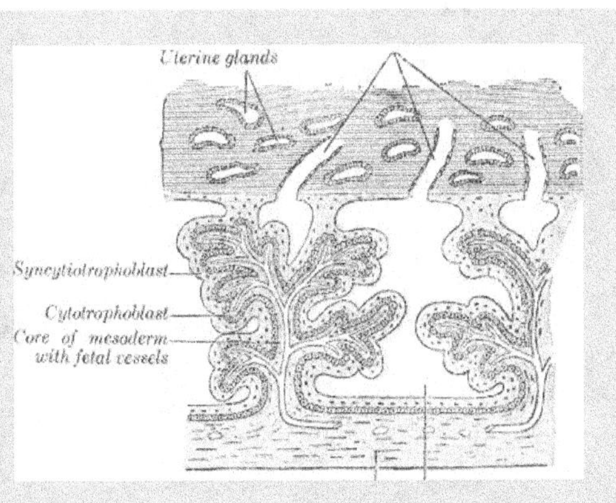

Placenta

Placenta is a highly vascular, disc-like structure by which the fetus is attached to the mother's uterine wall.

Placenta consist of two components:

1. maternal component
2. Fetal Component

Fetal component

- Develops from chorion frondosum.
- During development of placenta, small finger-like projections (called chorionic villi) arise from chorion to Decidua.
- Initially chorionic villi is found all around the chorionic sac. As the chorionic sac enlarges the chorionic villi in relation to decidua capsularis get compressed and degenerate. This part of chorion becomes smooth and is now called "chorion laeve "
- The chorionic villi in relation to decidua basalis grow extensively into decidua basalis, this part is called chorion frondosum.
- Chorion frondosum forms Chorionic villi, Intervillous spaces & Cytotrophoblastic shell

    1. Primary villi : Derived from cytotrophoblast and covered by syncytiotrophoblast
    2. Secondary villi : Mesodermal core (extraembryonic type) penetrates into primary villi to form secondary villi
    3. Tertiary villi : Mesodermal core develops fetus blood vessels. In this stage it is known as terminal villus.

Cytotrophoblast from apical region of villi penetrates the Syncytiotrophoblast to reach decidua basalis where it spreads out to form a layer called cytotrophoblastic shell.

Intervillous spaces are lacunae in syncytiotrophoblast, which communicate with each other and are filled with maternal blood.

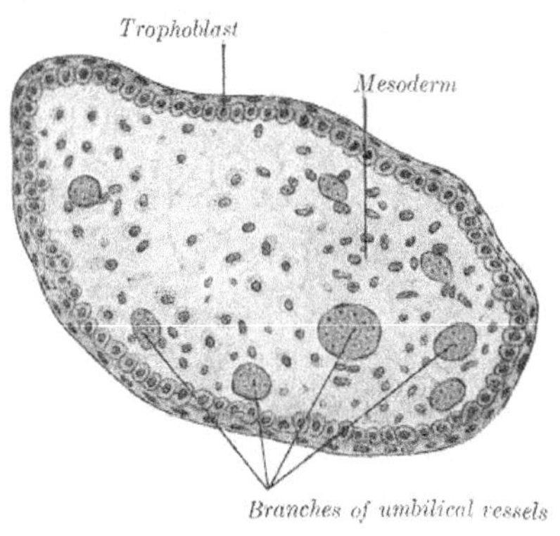

Img: Transverse section of a chorionic villus.

Maternal component

- Maternal component is formed by decidua basalis.
- Decidua basalis provides the site where chorionic frondosum grow to form villi and intervillous spaces.
- Decidua basalis also forms septa which grows into intervillous space and divides it into various Lobules or cotyledons.

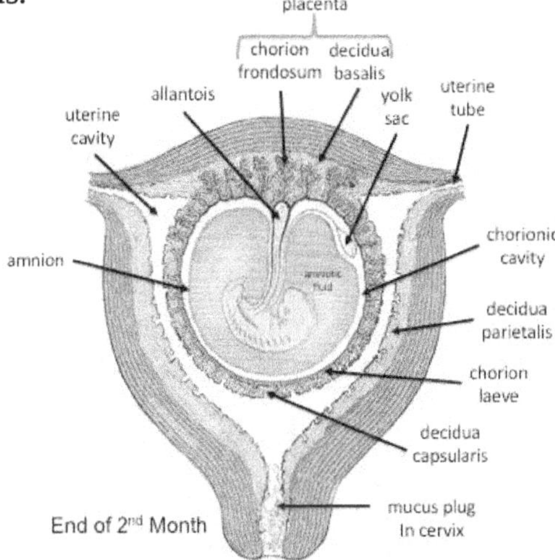

Img[6]: maternal and fetal components of placenta _image credit :Dennis M DePace, PhD, CC SA 4.0 via wikimedia

Full term placenta

- Disc shaped
- 500–600 gm weight
- 3cm thick
- It has two surfaces.
- Maternal surface – Present 15-20 lobules/ cotyledons
- Fetal surface – Provides attachment to umbilical cord

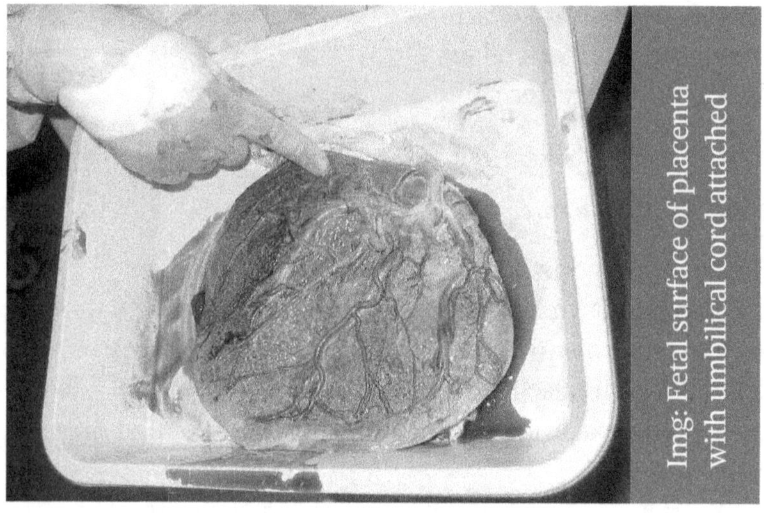

Img: Fetal surface of placenta with umbilical cord attached

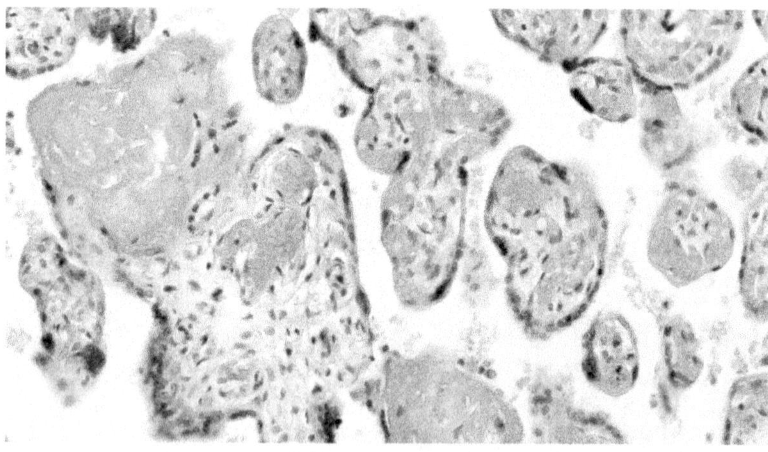

Img: Histological appearance of placental tissue

Clinical aspects

• Hydatidiform mole or vesicular mole:
- it occurs due to excessive proliferation of trophoblast which give rise to a vesicular or polycystic mass.
- This leads to the death of the embryo.
• Anomalies of placenta according to its shape
- Bilobed/bidiscordial - placenta consist of two lobes
- multilobular - placenta is divided into more than two
- placenta succenturiata - in this a small placenta is connected to the main placenta by blood vessels.
- Placenta fenestrata - In this, a hole is present in placental disc

(?) What is placenta previa (abnormal implantation of placenta)?
Ans: Implantation of Placenta in the lower uterine segment is called placenta previa
→incidence 1:200
There are 4 degrees of placenta previas:
1st degree - attachment of placenta does not reach up to internal os
2nd degree - Margin of placenta reaches the internal os, but does not cover it.
3rd degree - edge of placenta covers the internal o.s but placenta doesn't occlude the internal os
4th degree placenta - completely covers internal os and completely occludes it.
NOTE:
Painless bleeding in the 3rd trimester of Pregnancy is a diagnostic feature of placenta previa. It commonly occurs in the 4th degree of placenta previa.

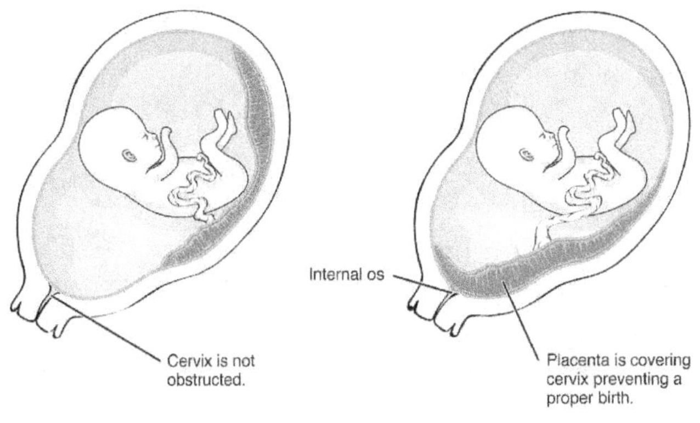

Img[7]: placenta previa grade 4 _img credit _OpenStax College • CC BY 3.0 via wikimedia commons

Amnion

- Is a thin, tough embryonic membrane that forms amniotic sac filled with amniotic fluid.
- Initially it lies the dorsal aspect of embryonic disc but as it later enlarges it envelops the embryo, future umbilical cord and fetal part of placenta.
- It completely develops during 10-12 weeks of intrauterine life .
- The amnion consist of 2 layers:

    1. Inner layer of amniogenic cells
    2. Outer layer of somatopleuric cells.

- Amniotic sac is filled with amniotic fluid.
- The composition of amniotic fluid – metabolites, hormones(HPL, HCG), cells of fetal epithelium, fetal urine.
- The amniotic fluid is formed by- filtration of fluid from maternal and fetal vessels, urine secreted by the fetus.
- Circulation of amniotic fluid- A part of it goes into maternal blood , a part of it is swallowed by the fetus, which is absorbed by the GIT of the fetus

Functions of amniotic fluid

1. Protects embryo from injury.
2. Permits symmetric external growth of embryo.
3. Allows the free movement of the fetus for the proper development of the musculoskeletal system.
4. Helps in the dilation of cervix during birth.

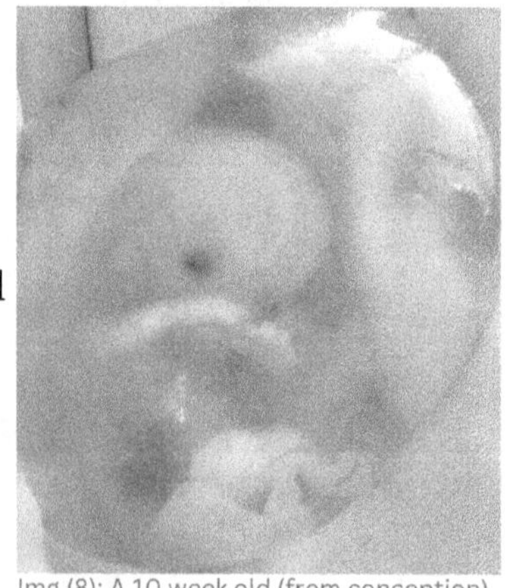

Img (8): A 10 week old (from conception) fetus in the amniotic sac (removed during a hysterectomy to treat carcinoma)
Img credit: CC BY-SA 2.0 author drsuparna

Clinical aspects

OLIGOHYDRAMNIOS:- the condition in which the amount of amniotic fluid is less than 400 ml.
Cause:- Reduced placental blood flow, renal agenesis, as a result pulmonary hypoplasia, limb defects, compression of umbilical cord.
POLYHYDRAMNIOS:- Is a condition in which the amount of amniotic fluid is more than 2000ml. Causes:- Esophageal atresia Or defects in CNS because of these the fetus is unable to swallow the amniotic fluid so amniotic fluid accumulated.

AMNIOCENTESIS – aspiration of amniotic fluid to detect the chromosomal abnormalities of the fetus. Done at 14 or 15th week of gestation. 200 ml of fluid is aspirated.

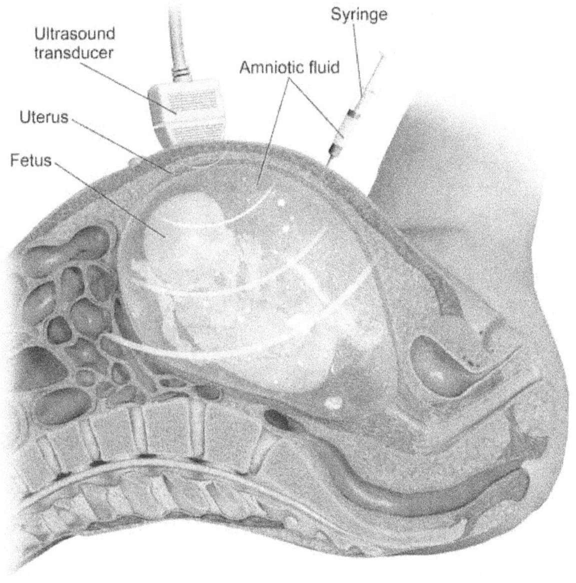

Img[9]: Amniocentesis CC BY-SA 4.0 via wikimedia author - BruceBlaus

Yolk sac and Allantois

It is an endodermal sac lying to the ventral aspect of the embryonic disc. It is a vestigial structure in humans. It passes through following three stages of development

1. Primary yolk sac
2. Secondary yolk sac
3. Tertiary yolk sac

Yolk sac has following functions

1. Hematopoiesis
2. Formation of primitive gut
3. Formation of primordial germ cells
4. Formation of allantois

Allantois is a small diverticulum arises from the caudal part of yolk sac during 3rd week

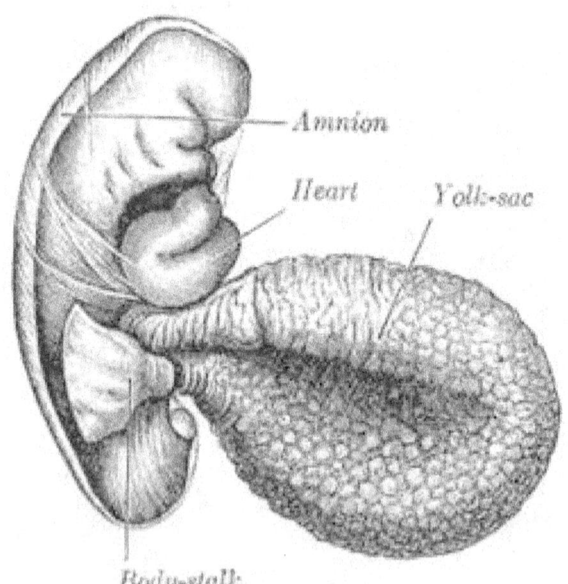

Umbilical cord

Umbilical cord is a cord-like structure by which the fetus is attached to the placenta. It is covered by glistening amniotic membrane. Contents of umbilical cord are

1. One umbilical vein
2. Two umbilical arteries
3. Wharton's jelly
4. Remnants of allantois

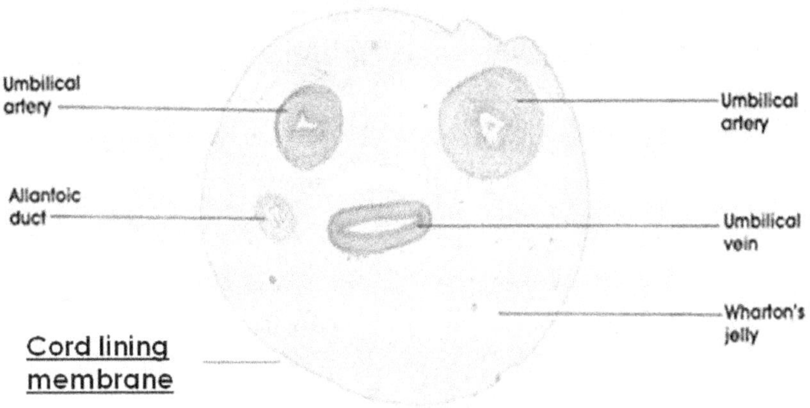

Img[10]: Cross section of the umbilical cord. Img credit_ Johnlancer123 • CC BY–SA 3.0

Development of nervous system

- The cells of ectoderm overlying notochord differentiated into specialized cells called neuroectodermal cells
- Neuroectodermal cells proliferates to form neural plate
- Margins of the neural plate get elevated as mesoderm proliferates on either side of the notochord. This leads to the formation of neural groove flanked by neural folds
- Neural folds moves towards the midline and fuses with each other to form a cylindrical neural tube
- The cells in the tip of neural folds do not take part in the formation of neural tube they are known as neural crest cells
- At 4th week the cranial part of the neural tube develops three distinct dilatations called primary brain vesicles. Craniocaudally they are

> 1. Prosencephalon
> 2. Mesencephalon
> 3. Rhombencephalon

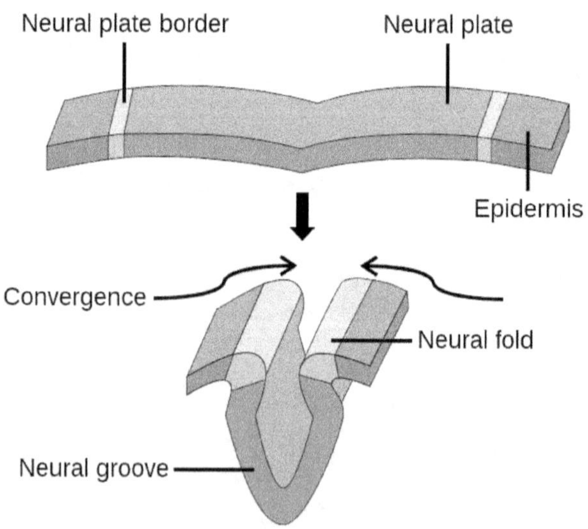

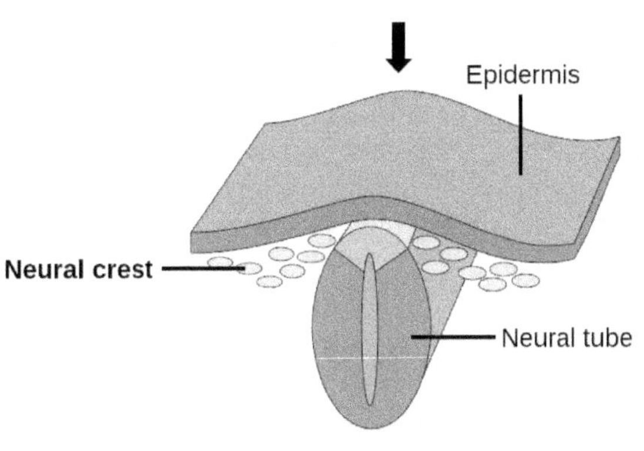

Epidermis
Neural crest
Neural tube

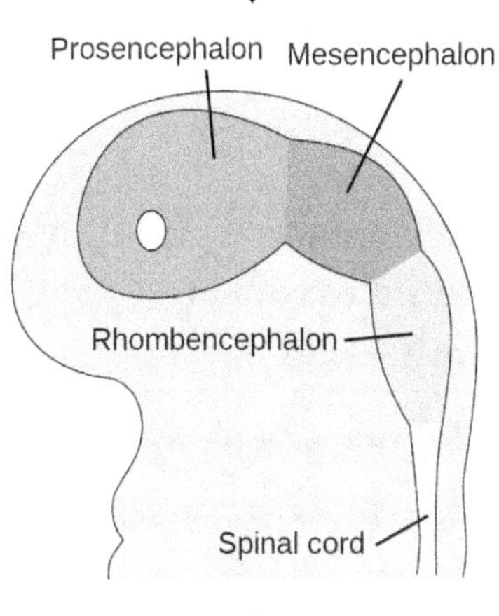

Prosencephalon
Mesencephalon
Rhombencephalon
Spinal cord

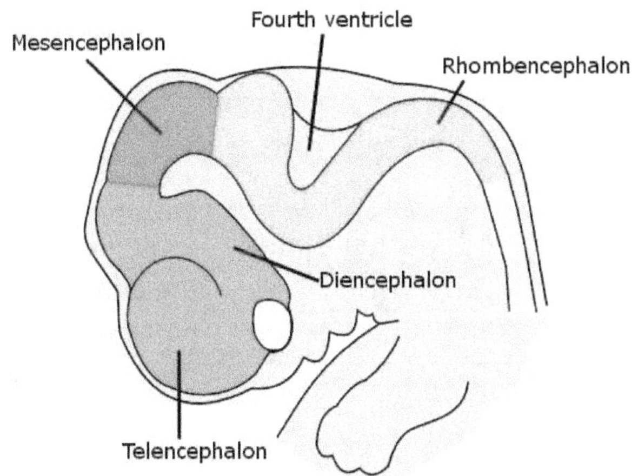

Mesencephalon
Fourth ventricle
Rhombencephalon
Diencephalon
Telencephalon

During 5th week prosencephalon subdivides into

1. Telencephalon
2. Diencephalon

And Rhombencephalon subdivides into

1. Metencephalon
2. Myelencephalon

Whereas Mesencephalon gives rise to Midbrain. So during 5 th week we can see a total of 5 dilations. They are called secondary brain vesicles.
The caudal part of neural tube develops into spinal cord

Primary brain vesicles	Secondary brain vesicles (during 5th week)	Develops into
Prosencephalon	1)Telencephalon 2)Diencephalon	1)Cerebrum 2)Diencephalon (including thalamus, hypothalamus, metathalamus, Subthalamus, Epithalamus)
Mesencephalon	Midbrain	Midbrain
Rhombencephalon	1)Metencephalon 2)Myelencephalon	1)pons 2)cerebellum 3)medulla oblongata

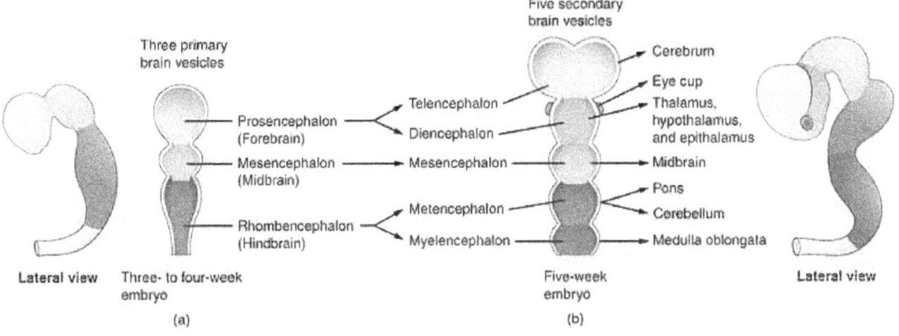

Img[11]: Derivatives of brain vesicles _ copyright OpenStax CC BY 4.0 via wikimedia commons

Derivatives of neural crest cells

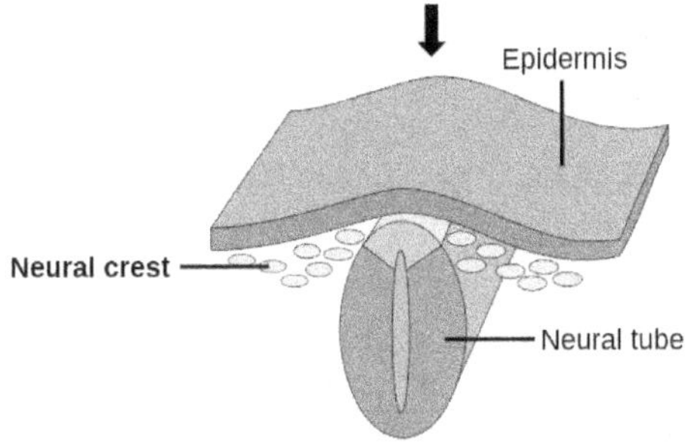

1. Dorsal root ganglia
2. Sensory ganglia of cranial nerves
3. Spinal ganglia
4. Melanocytes
5. Adrenal medulla
6. Schwann cells

Development of vertebrae, muscles and skin

Intraembryonic mesoderm on either side of the neural tube divides into 3 parts. From medial to lateral these are

1. Paraxial mesoderm
2. Intermediate mesoderm
3. Lateral plate mesoderm

The paraxial mesoderm undergoes segmentation to form somites. By the end of 5 th week, about 44 pairs of somites are formed in the human embryo. Each somite is triangular in shape with a slit-like cavity in the center. Each somites are divided into 3 parts they are

1. Sclerotome - Forms vertebrae and ribs
2. Myotome - Forms muscles
3. Dermatome - Forms dermis of skin

Lateral plate mesoderm forms body cavities. Where as intermediate mesoderm forms genitourinary system

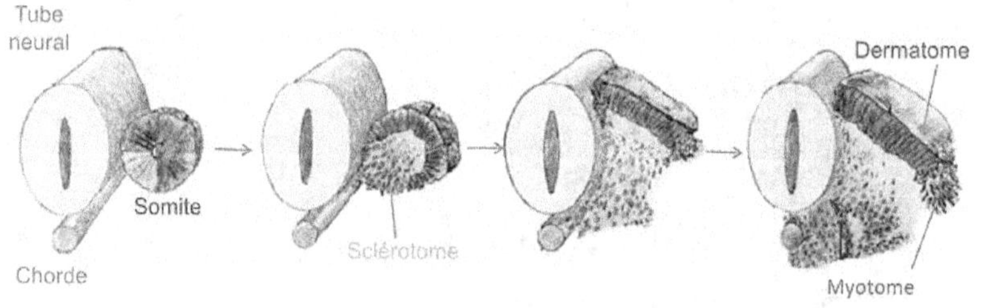

Image [12] : somites and its divisions image credit _Homme en Noir CC BY-SA 4.0 via wikimedia commons

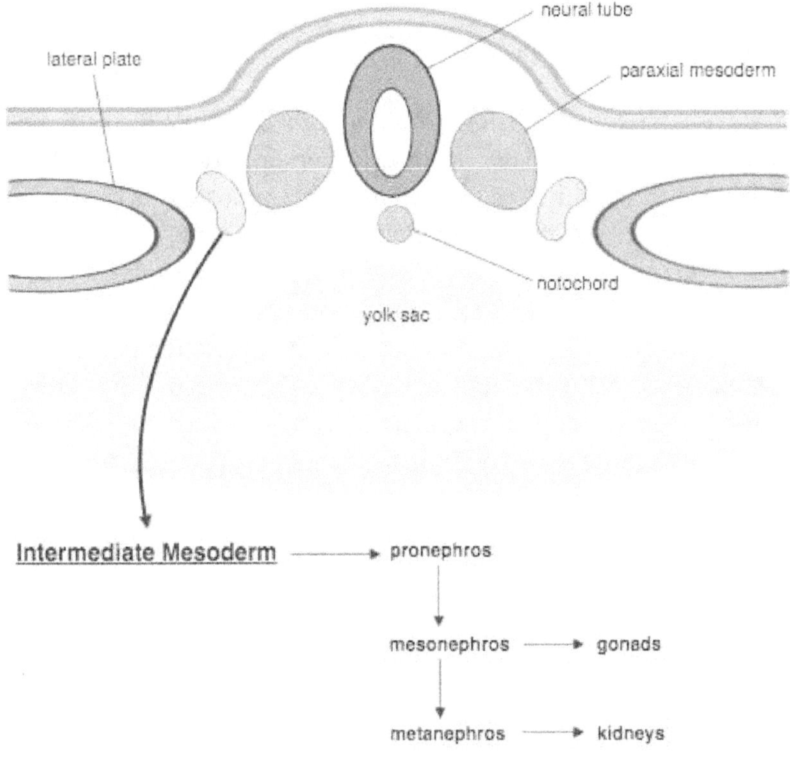

Img credit [13]: Jessica Xu CC BY-SA 4.0 via wikimedia commons

Lateral plate mesoderm forms body walls and body cavities. Initially it gave rise to intraembryonic coelom. During second month, the intraembryonic coelom is divided into three parts:

1. Pericardial cavity
2. Two peritoneal cavities
3. Pericardioperitoneal canals

Development of GIT

Primitive gut tube is formed from the dorsal part of yolk sac which is incorporated into the body of embryo during folding.During folding of the embryo, the part of yolk sac which is incorporated into the body of embryo develops into primitive gut tube. The part of yolk sac that lies (ventral part) outside the body of embryo is connected to the midgut by a narrow tube called vitelline duct.Vitelline duct connects the midgut to the part of yolk sac that lies outside the body of embryo. The primitive gut tube extends from buccopharyngeal membrane to cloacal membrane and divides into foregut,midgut and hindgut.

Foregut develops into	Midgut develops into	Hindgut develops into
1.Esophagus	1.lower duodenum	1.distal one third of transverse colon
2.Stomach	2.jejunum,ileum	2.descending colon
3.Liver,gallbladder	3.ceacum	3.sigmoidal colon
4.Pancreas	4.appendix	4.rectum
5.Upper duodenum	5.ascendingcolon	5.upper anal canal
	6.proximal two third of transverse colon.	

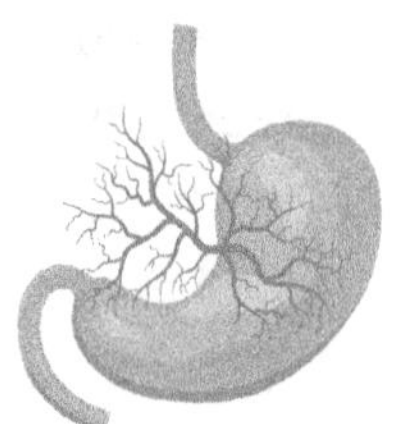

Artery of foregut is celiac trunk
Artery of midgut is superior mesenteric
Artery of hindgut is inferior mesenteric

Meckel's diverticulum

Meckel's diverticulum is the persistent proximal part of vitellointestinal duct(vitelline duct) which is present in embryo, and which normally disappears during the 6th week of intrauterine life.

- It occurs in 2 percent of subjects.
- It is usually 5 cm long.
- It is situated 60cm proximal to ileocecal junction.
- It is more common in men.
- Its caliber is equal to ileum.
- Its apex may be free or attached to the umbilicus, to the mesentery or any other abdominal structure by a fibrous band.
- It may contain ectopic gastric mucosa and pancreatic tissue

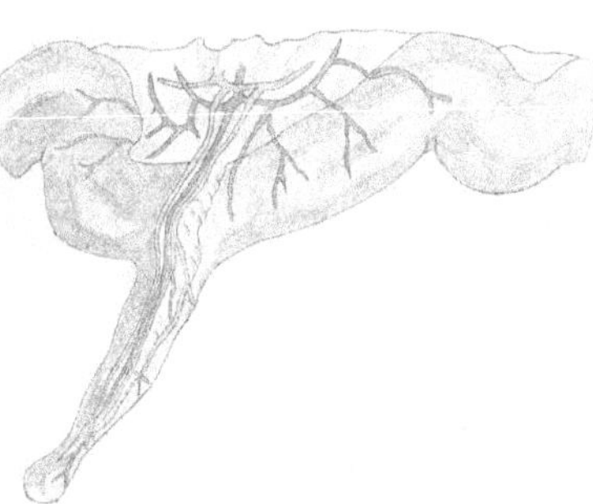

Img[14] : Diagrammatic representation of Meckel's diverticulum
img credit : Raziel at French Wikipedia. CC SA 1.0

Development of liver and pancreas

Liver develops from 3 sources

1) Liver bud – it is an endoderm derived structure arises from the convexity of duodenum. It subdivided into

- Pars cystica – give rise to gallbladder and cystic duct
- Pars hepatica – give rise to hepatic ducts, bile canaliculi and hepatic cords of liver cells

2) Vitelline veins – breaks into blood sinusoids

3) Septum transversum – forms capsule and hepatic stroma

Pancreas develops from ventral and dorsal pancreatic buds

Development of Heart

Mesenchymal cells in the cardiogenic area located ventral to the developing pericardial cavity condenses to form two cardiogenic cords. These cardiogenic cords get canalized to form two endothelial heart tubes. These heart tubes fuse together to form a single primitive heart tube. The primitive heart tube forms five dilatations.From cranial – caudal direction they are

1. Truncus arteriosus
2. Bulbus cordis
3. Primitive ventricle
4. Primitive atrium
5. Sinus venosus

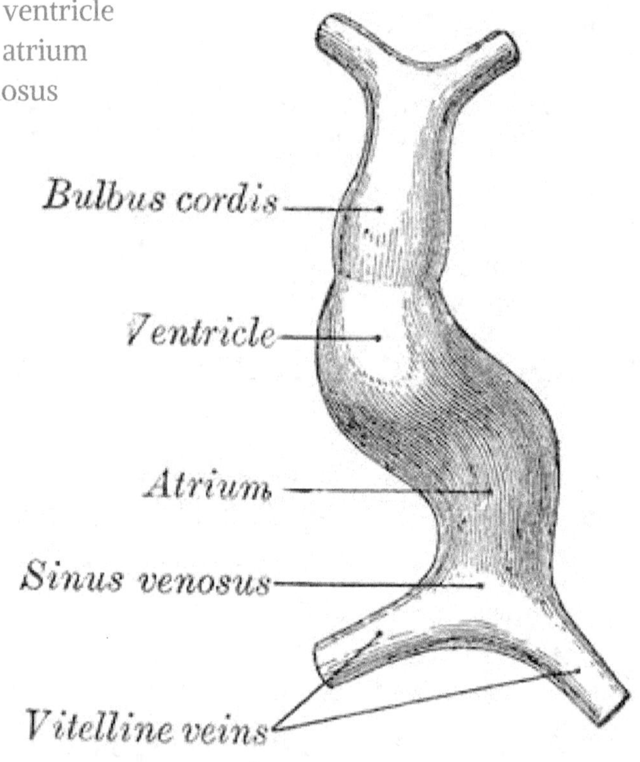

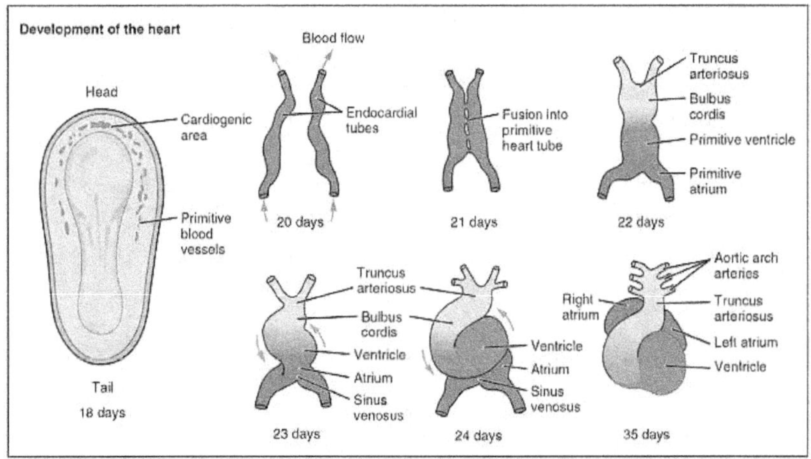

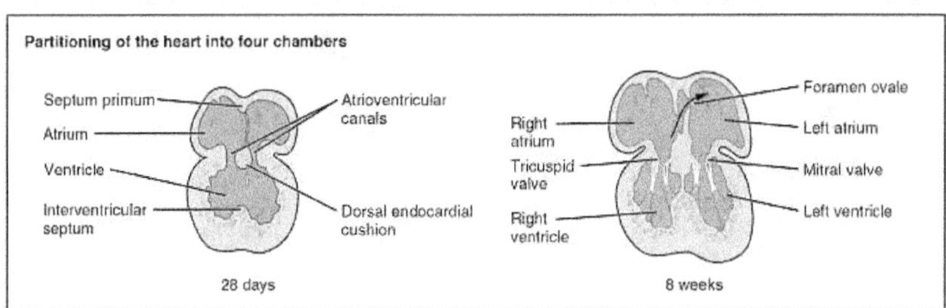

Img[15]: credit_ OpenStax CC SA 3.0 acess at Anatomy & Physiology, Connexions Web site. http://cnx.org/content/col11496/1.6/, Jun 19, 2013.

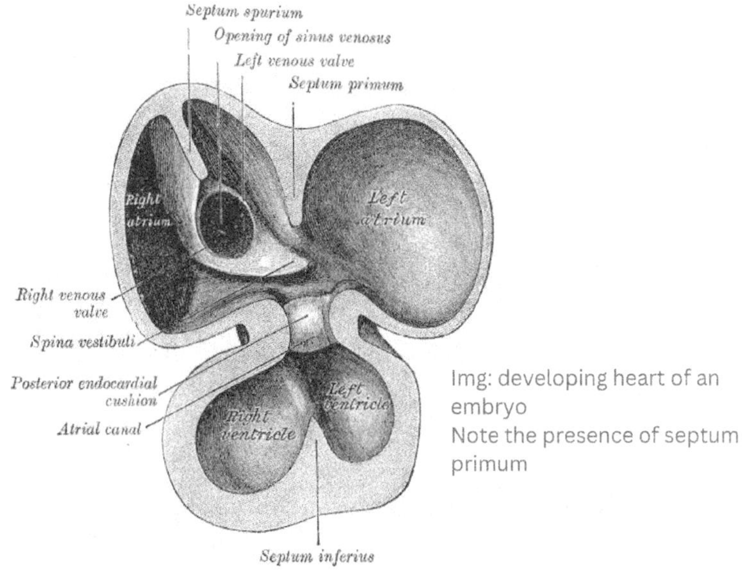

Img: developing heart of an embryo
Note the presence of septum primum

Part	Develops into
Truncus arteriosus	Ascending aorta Pulmonary trunk
Bulbus cordis	1) Smooth upper part of right ventricle(conus arteriosus) 2) Smooth upper part of left ventricle (aortic vestibule)
Primitive ventricle	Rough part of right and left ventricles
Primitive atrium	Rough part of right and left atria
Sinus venosus	1) Smooth part of right atrium 2) Coronary sinus 3) Oblique Vein of Left Atrium

Formation of interatrial and interventricular septum divides heart into 4 chambers

1. Right atrium
2. Left atrium
3. Right ventricle
4. Left ventricle

Interatrial septum is mainly derived from septum primum and septum secundum

Formation of AV septum

by fusion of dorsal and ventral AV cushions

- Muscular part – from floor of the ventricle
- Bulbar part – from bulbar ridges
- Membranous part – by proliferation of tissue from the right side of the AV cushions and from right and left bulbar ridges

- Septum primum starts developing from the roof of primitive atrium
- Septum primum grows towards septum intermedium (AV cushion)
- The gap between the lower end of "septum primum" and "septum intermedium" is called ostium primum.
- Septum primum fuses with septum intermedium.After the fusion,upper part of septum primum disintegrates to form ostium secundum
- Septum secundum arises from the roof of primitive atrium, right to septum primum
- Septum secundum grows towards septum intermedium and overlaps foramen secundum
- Gap between septum primum and septum secundum is called foramen ovale

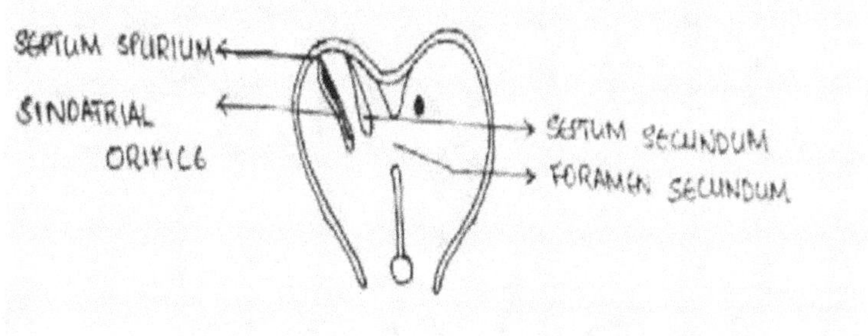

Development of arteries

- In the head and neck region, the arterial pattern develops mainly from aortic arches
- In the rest of the body, the arterial pattern develops from left and right dorsal aortae
- Aortic arches are six pairs and arise from the aortic sac. Each arch artery enters into the corresponding pharyngeal arches

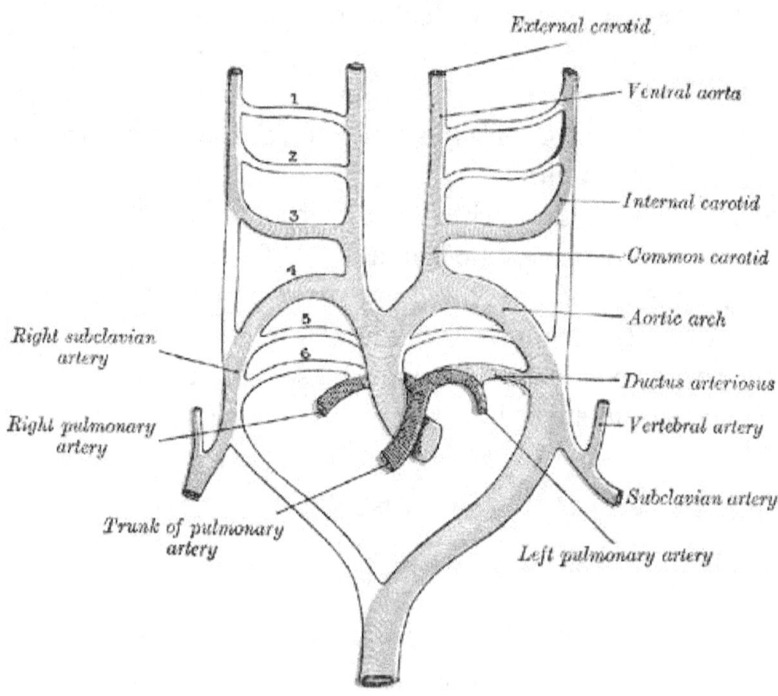

Arch	Derivatives
1st Arch	Maxillary artery
2nd Arch	Hyoid and Stapedial arteries
3rd Arch	common carotid artery and part of the proximal internal carotid artery.
4th Arch	<ul><li>Right arch forms the right subclavian artery</li><li>Left arch forms part of the arch of the aorta</li></ul>
6th arch	<ul><li>Right arch forms the right pulmonary artery</li><li>Left arch forms the left pulmonary artery and the ductus arteriosus</li></ul>

Development of urinary system

Intermediate mesoderm forms nephrogenic cords. This nephrogenic cords forms 3 successive kidneys

1. Pronephros
2. Mesonephros
3. Metanephros

Pronephros and Mesonephros are non functional and disappear. Permanent kidney develops from Metanephros and ureteric bud.

Development of ureter

Ureter develops from ureteric bud, which arises from wolffian duct

Development of urinary bladder

Distal part of hindgut is known as cloaca.Cloaca is divided into primitive anorectal canal & vesicourethral canal by a wedge shaped mesenchyme called urorectal septum.
Vesicourethral canal lies anteriorly and develops into bladder & urethra.

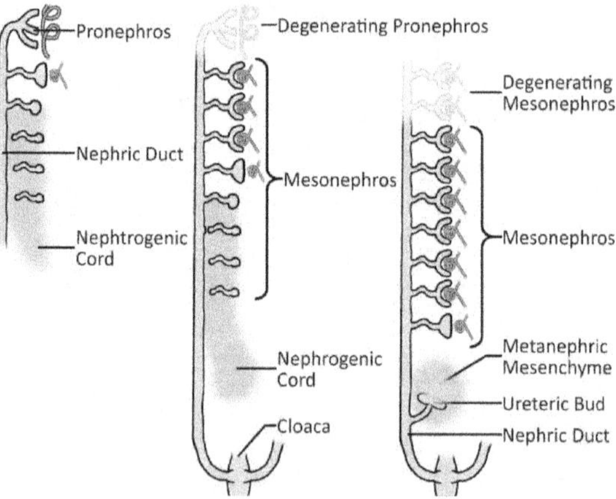

Img[16]: sequential development of kidney _img credit Ashley Sawle
CC SA 3.0 via wikimedia commons

Development of reproductive system

Genital system develops from 3 sources

- Intermediate mesoderm
- Part of cloaca
- Coelomic epithelium covering intermediate mesoderm

The development of genital system begins during the 4 th week of intrauterine life (IUL). Gonads do not acquire male or female characteristics till the seventh week of development; they are called indifferent gonads. From 7 th week onward development proceeds in different directions in males and females. Male gonads develop from Mesonephric duct or wolffian duct. Female gonads develop from paramesonephric duct or mullerian duct.

Male sex is determined by Y chromosome which codes for TDF (Testis determining factor or SRY). Male testis produces testosterone and MIF (mullerian inhibiting factor)

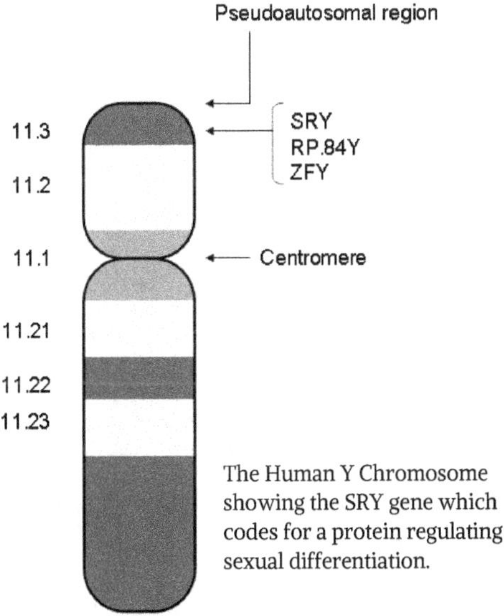

The Human Y Chromosome showing the SRY gene which codes for a protein regulating sexual differentiation.

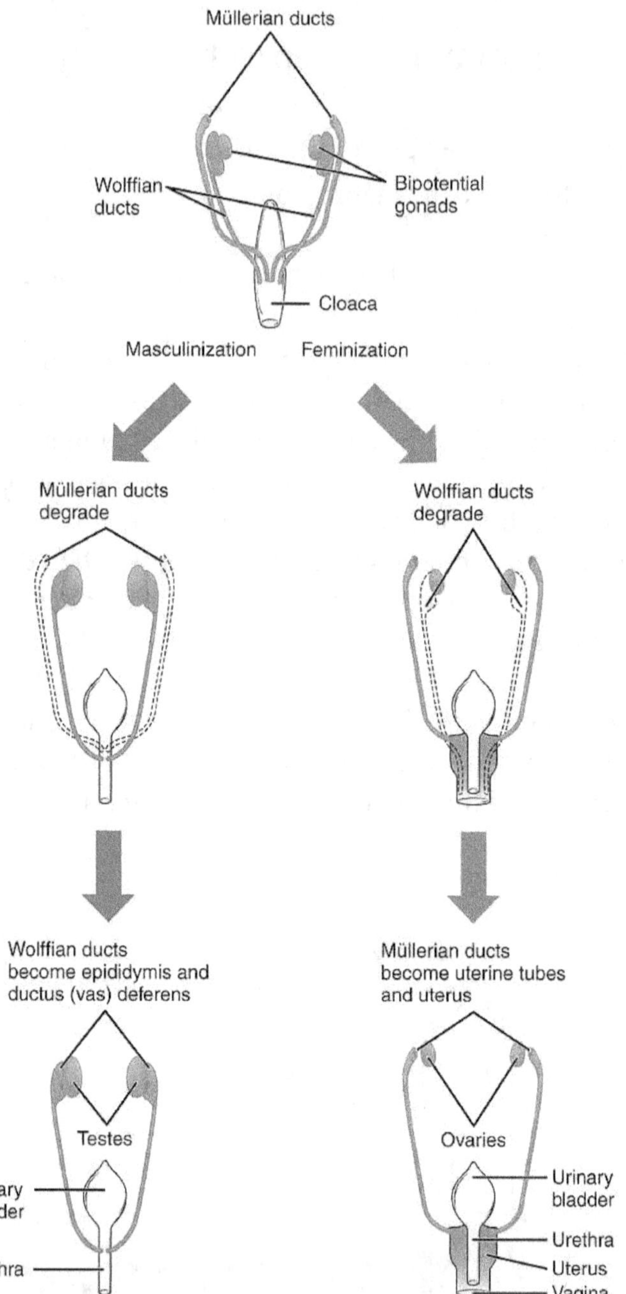

Img[17]: sexual differentiation in humans _img credit OpenStax College • CC BY 3.0 via wikimedia commons

Pharyngeal apparatus

Pharyngeal apparatus consists of pharyngeal arches, pharyngeal pouches, pharyngeal clefts and pharyngeal membranes. Pharyngeal arches are five in number (1st arch ,2nd arch, 3rd arch, 4 th arch & 6th arch) and present in the lateral wall of the primitive pharynx.

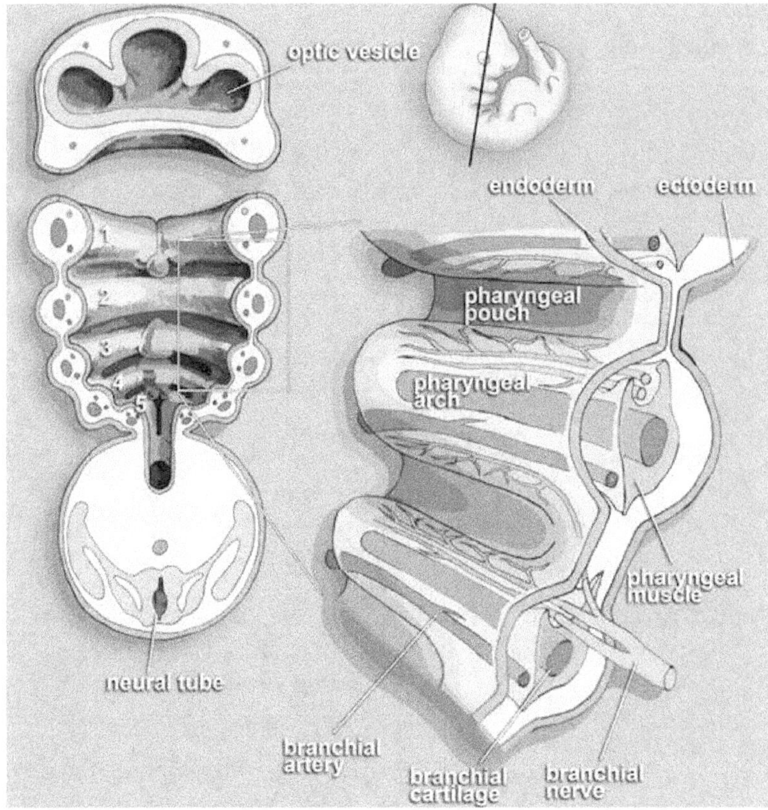

Img[18]:The scheme of the pharyngeal arches _img credit Loki austanfell CC SA 3.0 via wikimedia commons

Arches	Derivatives
First arch	<ul><li>Maxillary nerve</li><li>Mandibular nerve</li><li>Chorda tympani nerve</li><li>Muscles of mastication</li><li>Premaxilla, maxilla, Zygomatic bone and meckel's cartilage</li></ul>
Second arch	<ul><li>Facial nerve</li><li>Muscles of facial expression</li><li>Stapes</li><li>Styloid process</li><li>Lesser cornu of hyoid</li><li>Upper part of body of hyoid</li></ul>
Third arch	<ul><li>Glossopharyngeal nerve</li><li>Stylopharyngeus muscle</li><li>Greater cornu and lower part of body of hyoid bone</li></ul>
Fourth arch and sixth arch	<ul><li>Superior laryngeal branch of vagus</li><li>Recurrent laryngeal branch of vagus</li><li>Constrictors of pharynx</li><li>Laryngeal muscles</li><li>Laryngeal cartilages</li></ul>
Fifth arch	Regresses soon after its formation so no derivatives

Pharyngeal clefts are 4 in number. They are present externally between the arches

Clefts	Derivatives
First arch	External auditory meatus
Second arch	Obliterated
Third arch	Obliterated
Fourth arch	Obliterated

Pharyngeal pouches are four in number and located internally between arches

Pouch	Derivatives
First pouch	Middle ear cavity
Second pouch	Palatine tonsils
Third pouch	Thymus and inferior parathyroid
Fourth pouch	Superior parathyroid

First pharyngeal membrane forms tympanic membrane

Development of respiratory system

- Respiratory system is developed from respiratory diverticulum or lung bud
- Respiratory diverticulum arises from the endoderm of foregut
- Mesoderm lining the lung bud become visceral pleura
- Somatic mesoderm lining the body cavity become parietal pleura
- From the endoderm lining – larynx, pharynx, trachea and bronchi develops

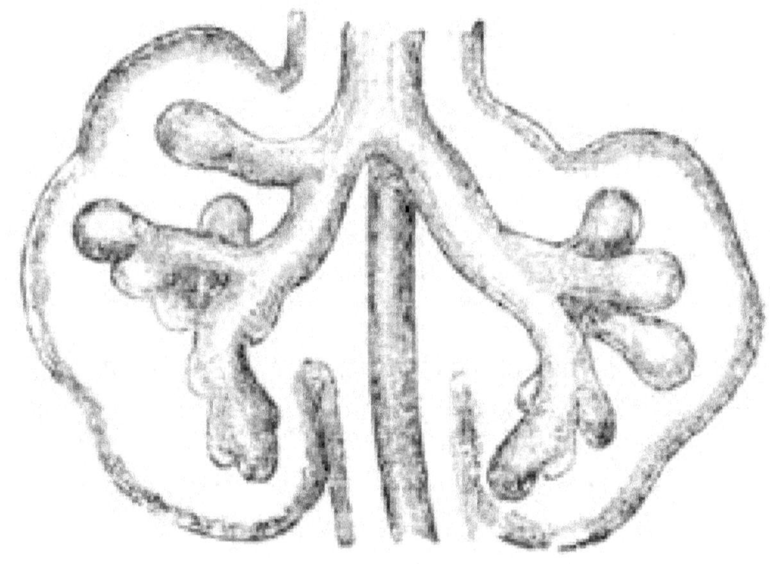

Img: Lungs of a human embryo at about six weeks

Development of limbs

Cells from the lateral plate mesoderm and the myotome (of somites) migrate to the limb field and proliferate to the point that they cause the ectoderm above to bulge out, forming the limb bud. The lateral plate cells produce the cartilaginous and skeletal portions of the limb while the myotome cells produce the muscle components.

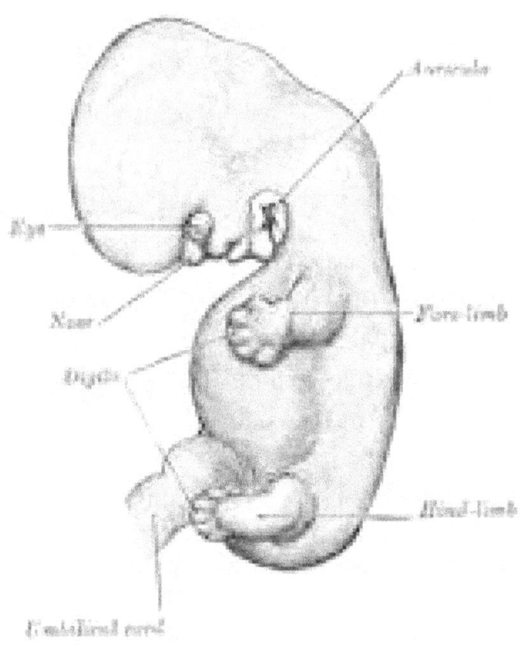

Img: Human embryo of about six weeks

Development of face, palate & tongue

The face develops from 5 mesenchymal processes which appear around the stomodeum (primitive mouth) they are:
1. Frontonasal process
2. Maxillary process
3. Mandibular process

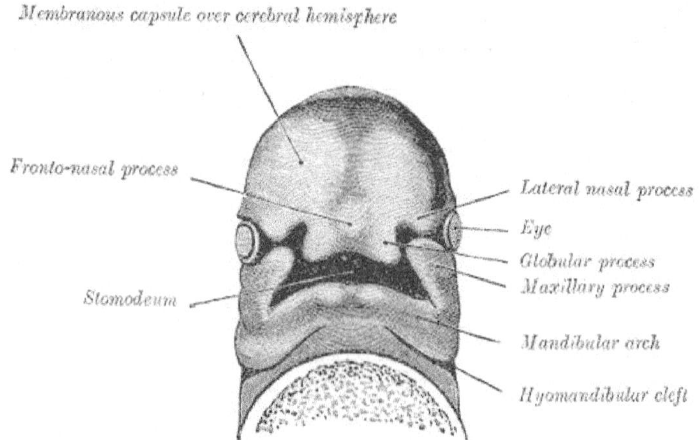

Development of palate

Embryologically the palate develops in two stages
1) Development of primary palate
2) Development of secondary palate
Primary palate develops from the frontonasal process
Secondary palate develops from maxillary processes

Development of tongue

- Anterior 2/3 rd from first arch
- Posterior 1/3 rd including circumvallate papillae – 2nd and 3rd arch
- Posterior-most part from 4th arch

Development of pituitary

The pituitary gland consists of two distinct parts
1) Adenohypophysis
2) Neurohypophysis
DEVELOPMENT OF ADENOHYPOPHYSIS
Adenohypophysis develops from an invagination of ectoderm lining the roof of primitive oral cavity called Rathke's Pouch. Rathke's Pouch develops in the third week of intrauterine life, later Rathke's pouch is cut off from primitive mouth or stomodeum. Anterior wall of Rathke's pouch proliferates extensively to form Pars anterior.
Posterior wall of Rathke's pouch remains thin and forms Pars intermedia. Cleft of Rathke's pouch remains as hypophyseal cleft which separates two parts.
A small extension of Pars anterior grows upward along the infundibular stalk and eventually surrounds it to form Pars tuberalis.

DEVELOPMENT OF NEUROHYPOPHYSIS
Develops from evagination of neuroectoderm of hypothalamus / floor of third ventricle.
The neurohypophysis differentiates into two parts

1) Pars posterior
2)Infundibulum
Neurohypophysis and Adenohypophysis fuse with each other to form Hypophysis Cerebri.

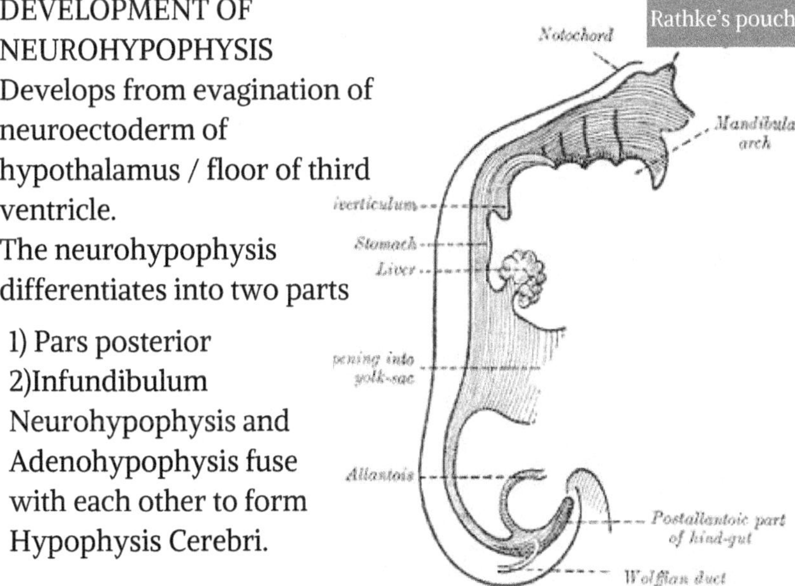

Development of Thyroid and Adrenal

- It is developed from the endodermal cells in the floor of pharynx
- It begins as a diverticulum called thyroid diverticulum
- This thyroid diverticulum elongates to form thyroglossal duct.
- The tip of thyroglossal duct bifurcates and proliferates to form two lobes of thyroid gland.
- Remnants of thyroglossal duct can present as

  1. Thyroglossal fistula
  2. Thyroglossal cyst
  3. Carcinoma of thyroid duct

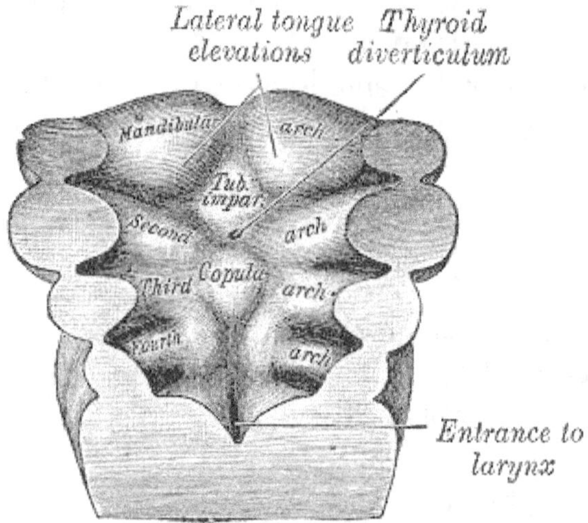

- Adrenal cortex develops from coelomic epithelium derived from mesoderm.
- Adrenal medulla develops from neural crest cells

Attribution

Img[1]: copyrt _Mariana Ruiz Villarreal _Public domain license

Img[2]: Image credit OpenStax College • CC BY 3.0 (Illustration from Anatomy & Physiology, Connexions Web site. http://cnx.org/content/col11496/1.6/, Jun 19, 2013.)

Img[3]:img credit: Leiladavids • CC BY-SA 4.0

Img[4]: credit _"OpenStax AnatPhys fig.28.2 – Sperm Fertilization – by OpenStax, license: Creative Commons Attribution. Source: book 'Anatomy and Physiology', https://openstax.org/details/books/anatomy-and-physiology.

Img[5]: copyright _By openstax CC BY SA 4.0] via wikimedia commons

Img[6]:image credit :Dennis M DePace, PhD, CC SA 4.0 via wikimedia commons

Img[7]: placenta previa grade 4 _img credit _OpenStax College • CC BY 3.0 via wikimedia commons

Img[8] : CC BY-SA 2.0 author drsuparna

Img[9]: CC BY-SA 4.0 via wikimedia author – BruceBlaus

Img[10]: Img credit_ Johnlancer123 • CC BY-SA 3.0 via wikimedia commons

Img[11]: copyright OpenStax CC BY 4.0 via wikimedia commons

Img credit [12]: Jessica Xu CC BY-SA 4.0 via wikimedia commons

Image [13]: image credit _Homme en Noir CC BY-SA 4.0 via wikimedia commons

Img[14] :img credit : Raziel at French Wikipedia.
 CC SA 1.0

Img[15]: credit_ OpenStax CC SA 3.0 acess at Anatomy & Physiology, Connexions Web site. http://cnx.org/content/col11496/1.6/, Jun 19, 2013.

Img[16]: img credit Ashley Sawle CC SA 3.0 via wikimedia commons

Img[17]: img credit OpenStax College • CC BY 3.0 via wikimedia commons

Img[1]:img credit Loki austanfell CC SA 3.0 via wikimedia commons

Your notes

Your notes

Your notes

www.ingramcontent.com/pod-product-compliance
Lightning Source LLC
Chambersburg PA
CBHW052235150726

48002CB00003B/1437